HEALING ARTHRITIS WITH CBD OIL

HEMP-DERIVED CANNABIDIOL OIL FOR RHEUMATOID ARTHRITIS

JAKE SIMMONS

Table of Contents

CHAPTER ONE

Hemp-derived cannabidiol oil for rheumatoid arthritis

In regards to CBD and Arthritis Pain, Here Is Some Important Information

The definition of cannabidiol (CBD) is not clear. Cannabidiol, or CBD for short, is a psychoactive element isolated from cannabis. While cannabidiol (CBD) won't get you high, it may make you sleepy. CBD is typically derived from hemp, a type of cannabis that contains 0.3% or less of the psychoactive compound THC.

Is CBD helpful for arthritic pain? Although CBD has been shown to reduce pain and inflammation in animal studies, these effects have yet to be confirmed in high-quality human studies. In anecdotal reports, some people with arthritis who have tried CBD have reported a reduction in pain, improvement in sleep quality, and/or a lessening of anxiety.

Is it ok to use CBD? CBD's safety is currently being studied in the scientific community. Very little is known at this time. Moderate doses have not been linked to any significant safety concerns. CBD may interact with other medications used to treat arthritis, according to some research. Patients taking corticosteroids (such as prednisone), tofacitinib (Xeljanz), naproxen (Aleve), celecoxib (Celebrex), tramadol (Ultram), and certain antidepressants (such as amitriptyline (Elavil), citalopram (Celexa), fluoxetine (Prozac), mirtazapine (Remeron), paroxetine (P (Lyrica).

Cannabidiol (CBD) products: are they legal? Hemp-derived CBD products are no longer illegal under the federal Controlled Substances Act because they are not considered Schedule I drugs. There are currently changes being implemented at both the federal and state levels that will ultimately clarify the laws and regulations surrounding the sale of CBD-based products. Despite this, you can find them in a wide variety of stores and on numerous websites. If you want to use CBD, you should research the laws in your state.

CHAPTER TWO

Beginning the Process

Is it worth it to try CBD? There has been a lack of high-quality clinical trials on CBD and arthritis, which has prevented doctors from determining who might benefit from CBD, in what dose and form, and who should be avoided. But there is consensus on a few key issues:

- CBD should not be used in place of conventional medicine when dealing with inflammatory arthritis.

To find out if CBD is right for you, talk to your doctor or other healthcare provider who has been treating your arthritis. What has worked in the past, what hasn't, what other options there are to try first, how to do a trial run, what to watch for, and when to come back for a follow-up visit to evaluate the results can all be discussed. Document side effects and medication intake in a journal.

• When used for an extended period of time, high-quality CBD products can add up in cost.

Make sure the product is actually relieving symptoms before shelling out the cash to buy it.

Which product should I look into more closely?

CBD oil and other products can be smoked, vaped, or ingested. Each has its advantages and disadvantages.

Through one's mouth. When taken orally, CBD is absorbed in the digestive tract. This is true whether the CBD is in a pill, a powder, a food, or a liquid. The delayed onset of effect (one to two hours), the unknown effects of stomach acids, recent meals, and other factors, make dosing difficult because absorption is slow.

Once a safe and effective capsule dose has been determined, they can be used daily. Edibles such as gummies and cookies containing CBD are not recommended by experts due to their unreliable dosing and the fact that they are appealing to children but do not come in child-resistant packaging. Medications in edible form should be stored in a locked cabinet, away from the reach of children.

Holding CBD liquid from a spray or tincture (a liquid dosed by a dropper) under the tongue (sublingually) for 60 to 120 seconds allows the cannabinoid to be absorbed directly into the bloodstream. The flavor might not be to your liking. The time it takes for the effects to kick in can range from 15 minutes to 45 minutes.

Upon the skin. Lotions and balms, which are considered

topical products, are applied topically to the skin over a sore joint. It is not known if these items penetrate the skin to deliver CBD. It can be difficult to tell whether the beneficial effects you experience are from the CBD in a topical product or from the menthol, capsaicin, or camphor that might also be included in the product.

Inhaled. A vape pen can be used to inhale CBD oil. Some people, especially those with inflammatory arthritis, may be particularly vulnerable to the unknown dangers posed by inhaling vapor oils and chemical byproducts. This, along with the fact that the CDC is looking into the possible link between vaping and an increase in the incidence of fatal pulmonary diseases, makes it clear that this is not a practice that should be encouraged.

What is the recommended dose of CBD for me?

Despite the lack of official clinical guidelines, the Arthritis Foundation has compiled the following recommendations from medical professionals:

• If you're using a liquid CBD product, you should know that the CBD extract is typically combined with a carrier oil, so in addition to the dose, you'll need to know how much CBD is in the liquid.

Stick to a slow, low speed. In the beginning, try taking CBD in sublingual form twice daily, starting with just a few milligrams. If you don't feel better after a week on the prescribed dosage, you should increase it by the same amount. Gradually increase over a few weeks if necessary. If you find that twice-daily dosing helps, that's what you should do to keep the CBD blood level stable.

• If you live in a state where medical or recreational marijuana is legal, and CBD alone isn't helping, you may want to discuss taking CBD in conjunction with a very low-dose THC product with your doctor. Keep in mind that even a small amount of THC can cause impairment in thinking, movement, and equilibrium. If possible, it is best to first experiment with products containing THC at night or at home, when you can sleep off any potential negative effects.

- If you don't feel better after trying CBD on its own or in combination with very low doses of THC, you might want to look into other options.

You should stop using a CBD product and talk to your doctor right away if you have any adverse reactions to it.

CHAPTER THREE

How to Find the Best Deals

There's logic in exercising restraint while out shopping. The sale of CBD products in the United States is largely unmonitored. Mislabeling and poor quality control have been revealed by third-party tests. The most common problems are mislabeled CBD potency, the presence of undeclared THC, and contamination with pesticides, metals, and solvents. What you should search for is:

Look for items made in the United States from domestically sourced inputs.

- Pick brands that adhere to good manufacturing practices established by the Food and Drug Administration for pharmaceuticals and dietary supplements (a voluntary quality standard because CBD products are not federally regulated under either category) or as required by the state in which they are manufactured.

- Only purchase from retailers who conduct quality assurance testing on each batch and issue a certificate of analysis from a lab that meets the standards set by the American Herbal Pharmacopoeia (AHP), the United States Pharmacopeia (USP), or the Association of Official Agricultural Chemists (AOAC) (AOAC).

Don't buy from businesses that make health claims about their wares.

Remember that salespeople in stores and on the sales floor are not trained medical professionals. That's why if you're going to use an unregulated product, you should consult with your doctor first.

CHAPTER FOUR

Rheumatoid arthritis relief: a review of the top CBD creams and products

For the most effective relief from arthritis pain, try some of these top-rated CBD gummies. Joy Organics CBD Gummies

Vertly Relief Lotion, the best CBD lotion for arthritis pain

• Lazarus Naturals Relief + Recovery Full-Spectrum CBD Balm is the best CBD balm for arthritis pain.

Top-Rated CBD Bath Salts for Arthritis Pain: Soothing CBD Bath Salts by Vena

CBD oil with the widest spectrum of benefits for arthritic pain: CBD Oil from Charlotte's Web That Contains No THC

LiftMode Hemp Extract Oil, the best CBD isolate oil for arthritis pain

Cannabidiol (CBD) has gained popularity as a treatment for a number of health problems in recent years. There is hope that

CBD, which does not produce intoxication, can aid in the treatment of pain, anxiety, and sleeplessness. People who want relief from these symptoms but don't want the psychoactive effects of tetrahydrocannabinol often turn to this alternative (THC).

Cannabinoids are extracted from the cannabis plant to create CBD products like oils, gummies, and creams. These chemicals could then be further processed into ingestible or topical preparations. Other cannabinoids like THC may be removed during the purification process.

CBD is an emerging component of complementary and alternative medicine. Hemp was taken off the list of Schedule I drugs in the United States in December of 2018. Because of this, research into the efficacy of CBD in relieving arthritis pain is scant. Although more research is needed, preliminary findings suggest that cannabidiol (CBD) may help alleviate joint pain without the adverse effects or addiction risks of conventional painkillers.

Read on to discover whether or not CBD products can ease your arthritis pain. Consult a cannabis-savvy clinician about the potential benefits of any products you're considering.

THE END

www.ingramcontent.com/pod-product-compliance
Lightning Source LLC
LaVergne TN
LVHW010513160826
845677LV00012B/2821

* 9 7 9 8 8 4 7 0 8 3 0 4 1 *